GO FIND OUT

a book of inspiration and call to action.

Dan Jones

iUniverse, Inc.
Bloomington

Go Find Out
a book of inspiration and call to action.

Copyright © 2010 Dan Jones

iUniverse books may be ordered through booksellers or by contacting:

iUniverse
1663 Liberty Drive
Bloomington, IN 47403
www.iuniverse.com
1-800-Authors (1-800-288-4677)

ISBN: 978-1-4502-3603-4 (pbk)
ISBN: 978-1-4502-3604-1 (ebk)

Printed in the United States of America

iUniverse rev. date: 9/28/2011

Contents

INTRODUCTION

Does God engage you throughout the day? At times, do you clearly sense His Spirit prompting you to take a particular action or respond to a specific situation, and yet you find yourself indifferent to Him?

Each time we turn our ear and our heart away from God's utterances and promptings, we render ourselves increasingly insulated from the Him. Before long, we are so immune that we can't relate to those who are open to the leading of the Lord. However, once you open yourself to God's presence, you will undoubtedly want more. And you can have more; just open yourself to Him.

As a believer in the Lord for more than thirty years, I've had the privilege and honor to experience many manifestations of God's glorious power and presence. Some of these experiences were nothing short of miraculous. With the utmost humility, I feel God encounters me not because I'm special, but because of His sovereignty and my openness to His utterances. The collection of super natural experiences and stories in this book represent a literal "whole other world" of events or occurrences.

This book recounts many personal experiences that occurred as a result of God's encounters with me. My hope is that anyone reading this book can look at my experiences and be inspired to seek a closer relationship with the Lord. It is my firm belief that these experiences will encourage you to remain receptive to the Lord's leading in your life. Through examples from my own life, you will *go* forward and *find out* His answers for your life's challenges. Prepare yourself to receive the blessings that will ensue from following God's Word and His leadings in your life. Together you have solutions to all of life's challenges. You will be able to walk in God's power through the fear.

ACKNOWLEDGEMENTS

To my sons Quincy and Noah: May we always celebrate the journey of grasping that elusive balance between ambition and acceptance.

The following folks provided the scaffolding for this project:

Kay Winer, my editor and friend: I owe you so much.

Charlene Jendro, my dear friend, supporter and encourager.

Lennon Tyson: Your grasp of the bible continues to astound me, not to mention your sense of humor.

The creative call class at The House of the Lord: You guys have no idea of how much you've inspired me; you are the best.

Terra Newsome: Thanks for your great insight and friendship.

The Diicypulz: Thanks for letting me use your music. Your music soothes my soul. I am so proud of you guys.

You, the reader: I pray I can convey my experiences and message as God would have me.

Jesus: You gave me the assignment; bless it and multiply it for your glory.

PROLOGUE

During the early 1970s I was best known as an instigator and activist on the University of Akron campus. Back then, descriptors like gambler, early stage alcoholic and hater of white folks were aptly deserved. Then almost overnight, I was transformed by God into a dedicated Bible-thumping Christian.

I was honorably discharged from the Army in July 1971. Shortly after that, I enrolled at the University of Akron. I was shocked to learn that the Black Studies program was non-accredited. Furthermore, the Black Cultural Center was a joke. It offered little in the way of cultural or academic help for students. To make matters worse, the man in charge of the program was completely incompetent.

Because I'm a person who is always looking for a cause, I attempted to address the problem. I ran for and was elected chairman of Black United Students' Community Affairs Program. I was serious about my job.

I immediately took on the school administration. I led protests. I disrupted stuff. I led student protest marches from the dean's office all the way to the president's office. On one occasion during a protest in front of the Dean's office, the police came and everyone ran except two white girls and myself. How ironic, since I was trying very hard to hate white people. One day I'd love to know the identiy of those girls.

What did I want? I wanted an accredited black studies program and I wanted a black cultural center with teeth.

Eventually I won, but at a terrible price. A university instructor warned, "Dan I applaud your actions, but I need to tell you something. You will never graduate from this university." I laughed. I had less than twenty hours to graduate. How could they stop me?

Here's how.

Two of my professors gave me a grade of F on my final exam. When I confronted them about it they claimed they lost my final paper, but they knew what grade I had earned. They would not produce my final nor would they consider changing my grade. They did however refer me to the dean. This is the same fellow that I had targeted for several protests. All he did was refer me to the president. The president was amused and threw up his hands in a manner suggesting there was nothing he could do.

I started to get the message. This scenario would repeat as long as I attended the University of Akron. In fact, I was informed that I should transfer to Kent State. So I quit.

I'm tempted to name names, but I won't. They know who they are and what they did.

As I mentioned, I did get what I wanted. I was even able to name the man that I wanted as Head of the Black Cultural Center. His name is John Wilson.

It was during this time in my life that God started drawing me. He approached me in ways that are not common amongst Christians. I had a conversion like Paul's.

One morning God told me to write his special message and my altered state of consciousness experiences in a book.

Go Find Out
A Spiritual Journey

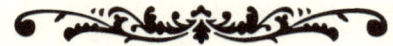

"Raise your hands high if you need Him
We operate on faith
We don't have to see His face
To say we've seen Him
We can't forget the one that freed us
So if you need a change
Simply whisper His name
Or call out Jesus"
Diicypulz—Mission, Movement, Music

CHAPTER 1

Who Am I?

I am an ordinary Christian with whom God has chosen to share extraordinary events. I have no idea why God would choose to manifest Himself to me in such startling ways. I certainly don't deserve it. I've made some awful mistakes in my life…some even on purpose. Yet, He forgives me and encourages me to continue on the journey towards sanctification.

I've not always been at peace with the notion of being an" ordinary" Christian. I'll never forget an exchange that took place at my father's funeral between a prominent pastor and me. This man of God approached me while I stood at the coffin viewing my father's remains. I was twenty-five years old and a new Christian. He asked if I was a pastor. I replied, "No."

He said, "Oh, are you a bishop?"

I replied, "No."

He continued, "Are you a minister?"

Again I answered, "No."

Then he said it —"Oh, you are just a Christian."

My head screamed, "Just a Christian." This man had no idea of the persecution I was enduring. He had no idea that I was being called names usually reserved for prostitutes because I refused to booze it up with my old army buddies. He had no idea that I was chairman for Black United Students at The University of Akron and that I was now learning to love white folks and being referred to as "Uncle Tom." He had no idea that guys were placing bets in the barbershop on the longevity of my walk with Jesus. Apparently the pain registered in my face and he offered an apology. This man did not even know that the guy in the coffin was my father...even though this pastor was officiating the funeral.

In any event, many years have passed since 1975 and I have learned that it's fine to be an ordinary Christian. In fact, when I read the Bible, I see God using ordinary believers all the time. Quite often, He uses them in extraordinary ways.

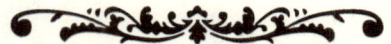

Praise God!

"And I know that
They don't really gotta receive.
And I know that
They don't really gotta believe.
And I know that
Nothing's new under the sun.
And I know that
We gotta finish what we begun.
Work all day to the very end
Work all day I ain't made a cent
Waiting for the moment I can finally win
Wake up tomorrow and I do it again"
Diicypulz 2009

CHAPTER 2

Why Write this Book?

I often think of people who never think of God. They are experiencing things that are difficult to describe, to believe, and certainly difficult to share. They are probably open to altered states of conscious experiences but are unaware of it. Not only do they encounter friendly forces, but evil ones too. They need to know that God often uses extraordinary devices to attract individuals that he wants to use for His glory. Often, these individuals are the least likely to succeed types or are even despised.

I write for these. I write to let them know that someone understands. They need to know that they are not crazy.

I also write to be obedient. Jesus gave me a message and told me to write it in a book. I remember thinking I had nothing to put into a book. He spoke to my mind to write about the experiences I have had.

You might dismiss the accounts in this book as some sort of psychological malady. Go ahead. One thing you cannot discount is the message. **Do what He says about your problems, particularly the most challenging ones. Tell me what you think.**

"We got to get clean
And get these things that keep us locked in darkness
Out of our lives and get seen
It's convincing
I'm just giving you the words that He gave me
And I pray to God you're listening."
Diicypulz—Mission, Movement, Music

CHAPTER 3

When God Gift Wraps a Message

Do little events play out over and over in your life? Are people in awe of you from time to time due to a special calling God has given you? If so, what have you done about it? Are you like me? Does God encounter you mightily ever so often? Does He, or His ministers, appear to you, speak to you, or protect you from dangers unseen but felt? Have you often pondered the meaning of these events? Have you taken the next step and asked God what you should do about them? I never did. But one morning God Almighty told me exactly what to do about them. He directed me to write this book.

Jesus has given me a special message for anyone who can hear it. A message that depicts how He helps us when faced with impossible challenges. It is a message so warm, so uplifting, and so fitting for a time such as this. Once you read it, you will no doubt agree that this came straight from Him. I have not read about it in any commentary. I believe **He gave it to me for those who struggle with being stuck. Those of us who are about to give in to that voice that belittles... that condemns...that voice that swears you can't do it.**

Imagine God Sharing a Secret with You

It happened about forty minutes into one of my devotionals. I asked God to give me something *fresh*. So, like many of you, I opened my Bible and was determined to read and/or study wherever it opened.

Honest.

Devotional time takes place in my prayer closet. It doubles as my

7

living room. Decorated with a black leather couch and recliner with matching cream love seat, it is very manly to be such a spiritual setting. With burnt orange, washed out painted walls, glass end tables and abstract art pieces mounted on either end of the couch, nothing speaks of femininity here. And just to be extra macho, the requisite 50" plasma commands center stage.

This Was Hardly Fresh

Mark, Chapter 6, is where my Bible opened. *"Jesus Feeds Five Thousand"* is the familiar subtitle. I chuckled and uttered aloud, "This isn't fresh."

I have read this portion of Scripture many times. I even facilitated a small group that focused on the events in Chapter 6, particularly the Scriptures relating to Jesus and Peter walking on water. However, to humor God, I decided to read on. Once I started, something miraculous began to happen. God was communicating another meaning to the familiar Scriptures. I felt him directing, encouraging and enlightening me as the Scriptures became alive. I was stunned. I cried. I was in another place—just Jesus and me.

God is No Respecter of Persons, but...

I can say with conviction that God gave me this message because of the devotional time that I spend with Him. I get to know Him during my devotion. I turn off my television and resist the urge to answer my telephone during this time. I find that solitude and silence are an important part of my spiritual discipline.

The True Love Litmus Test

God loves the time we spend with Him. Spending time with God shows that we love Him. Of course, you already know that. When people love one another they want to be together...a lot!

I recall a time when a very special lady told me she really liked me. I thought to myself, "this is great!" So I called her but she rarely returned a call. I emailed her but she would not respond to those either, at least not in a timely fashion. I even emailed her at work to no avail. Ironically, I have a friend who at this particular time had no telephone of any type. He had no car, no answering service, nothing. Yet, he stayed on the telephone with ladies. Half the time he was using mine. Here I am with home phones galore. I'm talking cell phone, fax machine, email, carrier pigeon and I can't move this woman enough for her to return a call. It finally dawned on me that this person really didn't care too much for me.

Now we know that God loves us because He gave his son as the ultimate sacrifice for us. We also know of His continual love for us because He is always thinking about us. Consider Psalm 139: 17-18.

> How precious are your thoughts
> > About me, O God!
> > They are innumerable!
> I can't even count them;
> > They outnumber the grains of sand!
> And when I wake up in the morning,
> > You are still with me!

So when you devote time to the Lord, you and He are having a love affair. During these times He often reveals treasures from His word.

It was during one such time that He revealed a part of this message to me. I consider this a secret because I have never heard it preached. The commentaries that I studied didn't discuss it either. So I concluded that it must be a secret. Does God have secrets? Will He share them with you? Absolutely.

When King Nebuchadnezzar was "wigging out" about a disturbing dream, he ordered the execution of all of the wise men of Babylon. Why? It was because they failed to interpret the King's dream. Of course, the King didn't give them much to work with. He demanded that they interpret his dream even though he refused to tell them the dream. How would you like to have a boss like that? You and the other top executives are hastily summoned to a meeting. The boss gulps and says, "Tell me the meaning of this financial riddle or you are all fired!" You reply, "Big boss man, this is highly irregular. Perhaps you could be so kind to tell us the riddle." To that the boss replies, "I can see through your trick! You are trying to stall for time because you know

I am serious about what I said. I'm trying to get something done here. Explain the riddle or else!"

Talk About Standing On Shaky Ground

Actually the wise men were doomed the moment the King issued the challenge. They were in a classic no win situation. Let's look at this. You read the King's mind. You also give him the interpretation. Now what? Every time you are in his presence he's looking at you and wondering if you know what's going on inside his head. You know what he did last night and with whom. Worse yet, you know how it went! What fate do you think is crouching at your door?

Remember Uriah the Hittite? He was murdered because a certain king didn't want it known that he, the king, was giving Uriah's wife, Bathsheba, the business. Kings lack a sense of humor about these types of shenanigans.

Whether they were able to tell the interpretation or not, they were history. The only exception to this is when God intervened on Daniel's behalf. Daniel's status as a wise man landed him on the hit list, too. God revealed the secret to Daniel who told Arioch, the king's executioner, not to kill the wise men because he would interpret the king's dream. Then Arioch quickly took Daniel to the king and said, "I have found one of the captives from Judah who will tell your majesty the meaning of your dream."

The king asked Daniel if the news was true. Daniel replied, "Your magicians, enchanters, or fortune tellers can't handle this but there is a God in heaven who reveals secrets."

Does God have a secret for you? Ask Him to share one. Open your mind and your heart because you are already hardwired to receive it.

"What's that name?
That name you was callin'
What's that name?
That you said when you was fallin'
That name is Jesus
Don't say it 'less you mean it"
Diicypulz—Mission, Movement, Music

CHAPTER 4

God's Message Under the Fish – The Secret Revealed

Let's explore a secret that God revealed to me in His word.

In the gospel of Mark there is a miracle that is known to many. What is unknown is the miracle under the miracle. Isn't that often Jesus' modus operandi? The more we fellowship with Him the more He reveals to us.

"Everything that is now hidden or secret will eventually be brought to light. Anyone who is willing to hear should listen and understand! And be sure to pay attention to what you hear. The more you do this, the more you will understand—and even more, besides. To those who are open to my teaching, more understanding will be given. But to those who are not listening, even what they have will be taken away from them."

The commonly known miracle is the feeding of the five thousand. **The unknown miracle takes place within that miracle. Mark 6:30-44 contains the story.**

Behold, When You Think You Stand...

The disciples had been out on what appeared to be a very successful missionary journey. They eagerly recounted what they taught and what they did. I have learned that times like these are when we Christians are the most susceptible to failure.

Witness what befell Elijah. One day he's on his high horse telling King Ahab, "There will be no dew or rain during the next few years unless I say so."

The next day he's running from Jezebel and asking the Lord to take his life for he was no better than his ancestors.

Were you aware that we are supposed to be better than our ancestors? I wasn't.

Take heed when you wear your pride like a jeweled necklace and your boastful words strut throughout the earth. Something just might come calling on your Achilles tendon.

As the apostles told of their exploits, a throng was pressing toward Jesus. There were so many people coming and going that Jesus and his apostles didn't even have time to eat. They left that area in order get away from the crowds for a while so that they could rest. As they approached the other shore, a throng of people eagerly anticipated their arrival.

People were actually running on the shore to intercept them as they landed. Jesus, though tired, showed compassion toward them and taught them many things.

Late in the afternoon his disciples came to Him and said, "This is a desolate place, and it is getting late. Send the crowds away so they can go to the nearby farms and villages and buy themselves some food."

Yes, it was getting late and the people should have been getting hungry, but did they complain of hunger? No.

Sometimes being in a desolate place is just where you need to be. In fact, I believe sooner or later, we will all log some time there. **When you do, remember human calamity is frequently a meeting place for God.**

Here is our problem and the beginning of the hidden miracle. People who Jesus is compassionate about need help. They need to be fed, but there is not enough food. In another gospel they said it would take 200 denarii to feed this crowd. One denarius was equivalent to one day's wages. It would take more than half a year's wages to feed this crowd. The disciples asked Jesus to send the people away so that they could buy food in the nearby farms and villages. Jesus said, "You feed them…" The disciples' reply was basically that it was impossible.

Dear people, when Jesus wants to use you for the furtherance of His kingdom, He first gets your attention.

He calls you…"You feed them." Who did they want to handle the problem? They wanted Jesus to send them away. Didn't they know He was the bread of life? Hadn't they just returned from casting out demons and healing the sick? (Mark 6:12)

Why did Jesus tell the apostles to feed them? Was He being an insensitive bully? I believe He wanted them to abandon themselves to the high adventure of following Him. **Recognize the full implications of knowing that with Him all things are possible, but apart from Him they could do nothing.**

Isn't it interesting that they had given up before accurately assessing the extent of the problem? Jesus says, "You feed them." Their reply is "With what?" Jesus asked them how much food they had. Then he told them to *go and find out.* After searching and taking inventory they said, "Five loaves and two fish." He then instructed them to have all the people sit down in groups on the green grass. He took the five loaves and the two fish and looking up to heaven, He blessed and broke the loaves. He kept giving them to His disciples to set before the people. He also divided the two fish among them all.

Did you catch it? If not, ask Jesus to open your eyes. Look: it's right there in front of you.

Lord Jesus, I pray for all who read this book. Open their hearts and their minds to the glorious opportunities you place before them during their time of desperation. Help them to behold your glory as they weep yet walk towards you with whatever they have to begin their process of deliverance.

For did you not say, "Come to me, all of you who are weary and carry a heavy burden, and I will give you rest. Take my yoke upon you. Let me teach you, because I am humble and gentle, and you will find rest for your souls. For my yoke fits perfectly, and the burden I give you is light."

Discover the Message

You are faced with an impossible situation. You are in a desolate place—a place devoid of resources. Perhaps the place of desolation is your marriage, maybe it's financial ruin or that you are living a lie and terrified that the truth may be found out. To make matters worse, it's getting late. The curtain is about to close. The shame of utter failure has no end. Life's desires have long since ceased. There is a consciousness that God has helped in the past but your heart laments that God has grown weary of you.

God's Help for Financial Woes

Medical bills, divorce, and sometimes just plain old poor decision-making have plunged many into a mountain of financial debt. If you live tenaciously in debt, bill collectors are in relentless pursuit.

Anxiety and bad debt are kissing cousins. They often result in dreading receipt of mail, and the opening of certain letters is out of the question. Even the strongest stomach turns and blood pressure elevates whenever that pink card shows up in the mailbox. You know, that card indicating that you have a certified letter waiting at your local post office branch.

You pray, "Jesus help," and He replies, "You fix it." You are immobilized, paralyzed by the enormity of the situation. Jesus whispers, "Go and find out." You wonder, "Go find out what?" Jesus whispers again, "How bad is it?" In your mind you know or at least you think you know. Abysmal—that's how bad it is! Your best thinking tells you it's hopeless. You have surrendered. You feel trapped. At first you are shocked that you are thinking of suicide, but later thoughts of suicide loom comforting. Yet Jesus still wraps His arms around you and whispers again. "**Go and find out** how bad is it. How does one do that? Yes, you must contact those very people you dread and discover all the itemized facts or information about your situation. Then you must explore your available options.

Here is the Key

Whatever you learn, take it to Jesus. Place it in His hands. He will gladly accept whatever little bit of ability and resources you have. He will bless it, break it into pieces (multiply), and give it back to you...you then pass it out and watch what Jesus does in your life. You, however, must pass it out. Praise God!

What does "pass it out" mean? You know, you must seize that very thing that is so foreboding. Get in touch with people to help you with debt relief, mediation and reconstruction. You must act in faith that the very thing you dread will move when you act in the name of Jesus.

16

Pass out any amount of payment you can. Call them. Set up payment plans. Revisit your values. What lifestyle do you really need?

Is Your Marriage Sinking

Are you starving for romance but your spouse could care less? You might as well be sleeping in separate beds. And don't you just hate it when they turn and roll away from you? Your heart grows suspicious. You cringe at the thought of infidelity and all of the issues that go along with it. You pray, "Jesus change my spouse." Guess what Jesus says? "You change them." You are gripped with fear. Sure, you may have seen miracles in the past, but Jesus doesn't know your spouse. Then Jesus says, "My child, you need to discover how bad it is and talk to your spouse even though you are afraid. Find out where your spouse is in the marriage. Maybe they are interested in counseling and if not make every attempt to open up dialogue. Your job is to unearth the loaves and fish. Perhaps the love remaining in your heart is like a mustard seed. Take that to Jesus and hand it over to Him with tears. Tell Him that this is all of the love that you can muster up for this spouse of yours. Jesus will take it, ask God the Father to bless it, break it into pieces and give it back to you to pass out to your spouse. This means any type of problem in your life, whether it be listening, sharing, counseling, debt resolution, problems with in-laws, or illness, to name a few. You must be willing to work with your spouse to improve and rebuild your relationship. You must act in faith and hold Jesus to His word, for He is always reliable. Watch and see what God Almighty can do in the life of your spouse.

Launch Your Talent

God has bestowed a special gift upon you. Be aware of how talented you are in this area. Perhaps it's art of maybe even writing. You can recall those blissful moments from the past when you were happiest while you were doing or enjoying your art.

Your life is a burden. Things are hectic. There are too many kids, too little time, too many demands and deadlines. You long for the day when you can just write, paint, play your instrument or compose your music. Do you sense that if you don't do it now you might never have the opportunity again because the years are passing? Emotionally, spiritually, and perhaps even psychologically, you are a mess.

What do you do? You know. Take whatever little time, resources, and inspiration you have and surrender it to Jesus. He will bless it, pray, and give it back to you multiplied.

You need to get busy and put Jesus in the forefront of your life.

Blinded by Success

You are a success. You are huge. You are a whiz at making money. Just look at how far you have come spinning wheels and making deals. And of course, the end always justifies the means. However, you are growing weary of the rat race. This intrinsic fear pervades. You feel that if you were naked or normal or struggling to make ends meet, people would not accept you. You loathe the trap you have set for yourself. It pains you that you can't mention the Lord at the office because you might lose the respect of your colleagues.

A voice whispers that there is more to life. Your family is in need of your attention. When you examine your conscience you realize that chasing money is the worst form of idolatry.

You pray, Lord, free me from this pattern that has trapped me. Oh, Lord to have a new heart and make a fresh start would be a dream. Jesus replies, "There is a way. Go find out what are the most treasured family times. However brief, small, or insignificant they seem, write them down and take them to Jesus. Give them to Him. He will ask a blessing of the Father, break it, and give the pieces back to you. You go and give them to your spouse, your children, or anyone who needs your attention.

Compromised Values Restored

Are you a young lady attending college? You say you love the Lord and you won't take it back. However…isn't there always a however? You are lonely. You are trying to serve the Lord but you feel like the only Christian left who has not bowed her knee to sex. Your loneliness urges you to hang around with the wrong crowd. You feel it's safe to go clubbing as long as you are just looking. A little window-shopping can't hurt, can it?

Along comes a hip, slick, cool dude just like I was when I attended college. Being good looking, I knew I had an advantage over the young impressionables. I hated professing Christians. I made it my mission to conquer their women by getting to know them in the biblical sense.

So there you are. You don't resist me. Not only are you rushed to the top spot on my list of hypocrites, but also your reputation is tarnished because I boast of my triumph to everyone who will listen. To add insult, you are the daughter of a prominent preacher. Your family gets wind of your indiscretion. Disgraced, you pack up and leave town.

What do you do? With all of that shame what do you do? When your life begins to feel shattered, bring any little bit of self –respect you can muster to Jesus. Take inventory of all of your good and special traits and ask Jesus to use you with all of your shortcomings—your warts and scars. Then entrust yourself to the Lord and walk in it. He will help you to see yourself and see things differently. Even the jerk that took advantage of your vulnerability will appear differently, although this may take awhile. Jesus will help you to see that when you change the way you see things…things change for the better.

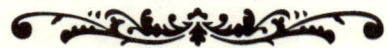

"In some ways we all fall short of His glory
But that's just another part to your story
I can read you."
Diicypulz—Mission, Movement, Music

CHAPTER 5

Army Times

In 1971, I was a paratrooper in the United States Army. I'm not boasting about being airborne. I just thought you'd like to know. You see, I didn't need courage to jump out of a perfectly fine airplane—courage was required to get on the plane. Once on board you're going out that door whether you want to or not. Big, burly, grizzly- looking jumpmasters made sure of that.

I was stationed in Thailand in 1971. My job was operating the Mars Station. I loved that job! You nosy types would have given your right arm for my job. Locating a clear radio frequency and making contact with an operator in the United States consumed most of my 7:00 P.M. to 7:00 A.M. shift. After exchanging pleasantries with him (it was always a him), I would check the waiting list to see who wanted to call home.

The Mars Station Was a Happening Spot

Soldiers desirous of calling home would call the station during the day shift and request to be placed on the call list. Remember, this was before the advent of the Internet. The list was always prioritized. Officers were first. They always pulled rank, except on my watch. I routinely called the grunts first and put through their calls. The conversations made for good entertainment and diversion.

The calls consisted primarily of GIs wanting to know about their kids and sweetie. Sweeties wanted to know if their GI had contracted anything mightier than a cold. Every now and then I would have to referee fights and enforce the no cussing rule. I derived much satisfaction from my role as sheriff. The reason I had to listen in on these calls was because I had to flip a switch when my party was through speaking. They would say "over" letting me and the other ham operator know when to let the other person speak. There were actually two of us listening in on these conversations.

My station was positioned on top of a very large hill. In the middle of the night, while working alone and unarmed, I often wondered how easy it would be for a North Vietnamese soldier to traipse across Laos, roll up on me and stab me in the back of my neck, bust me upside the head with the butt of his AK47, hang me upside down and split open my gut, catch the drops of blood in his helmet and...well, you get my drift. It was often very scary to be up on that mountain alone.

Thailand Was A Grunt's Dream

Yes, I admit that this was good duty, as we say in the military. I was stationed in a beautiful country on the gulf of Thailand with lovely beaches, gorgeous sunsets, and a sensual blue sky that at times I felt I could reach up and touch. No self respecting GI could describe Thailand without at least a few words about the women. They were lookers. Honest. Simply the most beautiful women I have ever laid eyes on.

I was a hit with them. I took the time to learn to speak their language. They were amazed that I could converse in something beyond soldier speak. You know, how much, how long, and can I see your updated medical card please.

My stint in the hospital afforded me the opportunity to learn to speak Thai. I spent time in the hospital recovering from a cyst in my hinder parts. It was as painful as it was boring. My Thai nurse saw me reading a *"How to Speak Thai"* book and offered her assistance. She delighted me. She was gorgeous, but beyond that she took a keen interest in my daily progress. The hospital was situated on Utapo Air Base where my daily activities alternated between reading my book and watching B-52's take off, presumably to bomb targets in North Vietnam. It took about a month to fully recover. Thanks to my devoted nurse, I was discharged from the hospital with a smattering of a lovely language.

Thais, both men and women, were impressed that I had taken the time to honor them by learning their language when most of them were trying very hard to master English.

The Call Begins

My introduction to miracles happened in Thailand. My cake job as Mars operator had another benefit- my work schedule. Alternating three days on and three days off assures lots of free time. One mid-morning I went to the grunt's club to play the slot machines. After losing all of my quarters, a stunning young lady entered the room and walked right up to me. She paused for a moment asking if I was playing this machine. I was down to my last quarter so I told her that I would be finished real soon. She waited and watched. I lost. She smiled and pulled a quarter from her purse and put it into the machine. Bang! Jackpot! I watched incredulously. She just looked at me and smiled. No one was in the room other than the two of us. She continued to peer at me with this incredible look. It was as though she was looking right through me. She asked me if I wanted to go for a ride with her. I was awestruck by this woman. The normal GI juices weren't flowing. I was not entertaining thoughts of getting to know her biblically; I was transfixed by her grace, beauty, and my good fortune. I agreed to go for a spin with her.

Parked outside was this huge car that would remind you of something you'd find in a presidential motorcade. The vehicle belonged to her. The driver exited and opened the door for me. My head was spinning— questions, questions, questions. Who is this lady and why is she taking me with her, me of all people? She uttered something to the driver in Thai that I did not understand. She turned to me and said we were going to Sadahipp to shop. Upon arriving at the gates the guards walked toward us, saw her, stopped dead in their tracks and waved us through. She offered to buy me a number of items as we shopped. I refused them all. She was so elegant. People nodded at her with the utmost respect as they walked past us. She made no purchases; she merely browsed and smiled at passers-by. I learned that she had studied in San Francisco and that she was the kindest soul I had ever met.

She took me back to the post after about an hour of shopping. The driver pulled to the club. She smiled as I got out. I managed a thank you and never saw her again. I went to that club the same day and time for weeks. No one in the club had any idea of this mystery woman. My investigation yielded nothing.

To this day I often wonder about her. How could she win that jackpot with just one single quarter? How could she look through me and yet gaze upon me so compassionately? And why did she never come back?

God drew me to himself primarily through love. This was my first taste of it. I didn't know it then but I do now.

"I had a change in my mindset
I had to go rearrange in my mind
I couldn't stay in that mindset
I had to make a change
Now I'm praying everyday
That He stays in my mindset"
Diicypulz—Mission, Movement, Music

CHAPTER 6

The Revelations Begin

A distaste for saluting officers was responsible for my being jettisoned from a cushy job in Thailand to the cold, rugged winters of Korea. It all happened as a result of me not saluting an officer correctly. I think my fingers were crossed or something and I really didn't care. I mean, at least I acknowledged his rank. He was not amused. Almost the next day I was on a plane headed for Korea. That officer must have had more rank than I realized. It's funny that with only 90 days left in the Army I was being shipped to Korea. Does that make any sense whatsoever? Was I key to some vital mission? Was my job classification top secret? I'll bet you are just dying to know what job I landed after brushing the snow off my khakis. I was assigned to the supply room. I counted sheets. Unless you insert God into this mess, you will be scratching your head for quite a while. God Almighty had plans for me. It was in Seoul, Korea that my encounters with God began in earnest.

God In A Storm

Leaving the movie theatre and heading to my favorite bar, I noticed dark, foreboding clouds rolling in. Storms materialize out of nowhere in Korea. During monsoon season this occurs frequently. In respect for Mr. Monsoon I quickened my pace. My concern was minimal because the club sat only a half-mile away. I was about one-eighth of a mile from my destination when lightening struck the power lines hanging directly above my head. They fell immediately at my feet. Energy and power engulfed me. Brilliant colors enveloped me. I walked right through them. Entering the club proved quite a spectacle. People stopped and

27

stared, actually some were downright gawking at me. I walked into the men's room for whatever reason. A look into the mirror revealed a man with hair spiking due north. Though I appeared disheveled, I was unharmed. There was not a singe mark on me. It didn't dawn on me as to what had transpired. My mind was elsewhere. After a couple of hours I was back to my old self—toasting drinks, dancing with the ladies, and engaging in the usual antics that GIs pull.

Mind Numbing Celebration

Duty in Korea was different—very different. In our hooch, celebratory parties were the norm. Any excuse to party was welcomed and wholeheartedly embraced. We partied because of sunny days. We partied because of rain. We partied because someone in a nearby company was short. They didn't even have to be in our company. A full moon always chipped in. And of course, no one's birthday escaped our attention.

It had been a long night of drinking. Upon my arrival back to our hooch a guy greeted me with a drink. Drinks were fine. Booze defined me. I was a drinker, not a druggie. Chemical users are crazy. Everything I drank had a color to it and it was usually brown. So it was with some suspicion that I eyed this particular concoction. It was clear. I hesitated and inquired about its contents. The guy (who was toasted) reassured me that it was cool. So like Adam I ate it. He offered another. I ate it again. Just a few minutes later my world changed forever.

Vivid colors exploded all around me. Streamers of red, orgasmic orange, hippie yellow, and brilliant blue shot through the night sky as I walked outside. This was weird but I loved it. After a couple of minutes I went inside, took a seat, and began mellowing out with the other guys, all of whom were sitting around feeling buttered. Suddenly events took a serious turn for the worse. Our company dog was sitting in the middle of us. Our eyes met, and then all of his bowels spilled out on the floor. He snarled at me with teeth flashing. Terror took over. I said to one of the brothers, "Hey, man I can't handle this." He gave me a hand motion signaling to get out of here. He said, "Ah, man you can handle it." But I couldn't. I jumped up and went outside to see more of the brilliant streamers. They never returned. Instead, hideous looking creatures appeared.

Flaky To The Rescue

Then a voice from beside me said, "Jones, what's going on?" I looked and it was Flaky. He was a white guy who had a reputation for partying. He was always high, about to get high, or coming down from a high. He and I were not friends or even good acquaintances. However, for some reason he was there. In my state of mind I cannot describe his mental state. I knew only that he cared. I finally answered his question, "Flaky, I'm seeing monsters, man."

He said, "Jones, if you look at them and smile they will vanish like poof, presto they're gone." Not believing him I shunned his advice. I just knew if I could regain control of my mind that I would be all right. What I didn't know was that I had ingested a hallucinogen that was tripping me out of my mind. I had never tripped before. I had only heard about them. I was a boozer, far too sophisticated to do dope. I later learned that our mind has a mechanism that differentiates between stimuli, and during drug-induced trips, that mechanism is turned off. The bottom line is whatever is in your subconscious will probably become your reality. I guess I must be a fairly spooky person…no pun intended for those of you who are still racially challenged.

I remember telling myself that if I could just remember the words to a famous song I would be fine. I tried to sing one of Michael Jackson's songs but the lyrics eluded me.

Flaky suggested we take a walk, so off we went. During our walk, my head appeared to disengage and stare directly at me, every fiber in my body screamed, and screamed, and screamed. Words cannot describe the terror of not being able to control visualizations, particularly when they appeared within inches of my face. It was then that I capitulated, deciding to listen to Flaky. With all of my might I forced a smile at this ghastly creature who seemed to double dare me to look at him. Understandably, I had been turning my head and covering my eyes. Finally, I managed a smile. Flaky was right! The ghastly vision disappeared—poof! I mean instantly. Each time another one would appear. I would yell to Flaky, "Flaky, I see another one!" He'd reassure me it too would poof away if I would smile at it. Once again it worked. Flaky was the man!

He then hailed a cab and we rode around for a couple of hours. Monsters continued to appear but Flaky's script worked flawlessly. As my confidence grew, they became less and less frequent. When we returned to base, Flaky insisted I hang with him the next day. I was a short timer; I had only about five days left before catching the iron bird back to the U.S. to be honorably discharged from this man's army. All that means is that I had no job. I had already cleared post in Korea so I was free to go with Flaky.

On my way to my room I saw the company dog and I was mortified. His bowels didn't spill out; I just had this intense fear of him. That fear didn't leave me for a couple of years.

The very next morning, Flaky and I hit the road. He picked me up in his deuce and a quarter. He was an Army truck driver. We drove all over the south of Korea. We neither delivered nor picked up anything. I didn't really know what his job duties were but he seemed to enjoy just riding around. Every now and again we would stop at a building. Flaky would run in and return in a few minutes. We did this for several hours. From time to time he would inquire as to my mental status. He knew better than to leave me to myself for very long because I was still in and out of my trip. It was not as drastic as the night before.

I feel that I owe my life to Flaky. I never got his address before I left. I don't even know his real name. All I know is that he saved me during the summer of 1971 in Korea. He was one kind man. I would love to meet him one day and thank him for all of the time he spent with me. I would also love to know just what his job duties really were.

As I reflect on that awful night of tripping, I recall one seemingly insignificant event. At one point I said, "God, if you will help me I will believe in you". I did not understand the magnitude and implications of that statement. I do know that God helped me. He sent Flaky.

This event did not lead directly to my salvation. There would be more powerful and frightening events to come. I do admit though that I always felt this nudge to remember how I asked God to help me and how the brothers in my company just blew me off. Yet God saw fit to send a white guy after me to look out for me. Flaky kept me from injuring myself while fleeing from monsters or jumping off one of those high hills that we walked that night.

"You might not know me
But you know what defines me
Still in the church so you know where to find me
Gotta save the world so you know why I'm crying
Gotta get to heaven
Oh you need not remind me"
Diicypulz—Mission, Movement, Music

CHAPTER 7

Church Stuff

After my discharge from the Army in 1971, I landed a job as an outreach worker for our YMCA. My job description insisted that I find kids on the fringes of the criminal justice system and intervene. I was responsible for making a difference in their lives.

While holding this job I met two young men, Michael and Alan, whom God used to change my life. They were participants in this group of kids I had managed to put together. Most of them attended Buchtel High School. These were not bad kids; they just needed something to do. They eagerly joined my group because I promised we'd do stuff.

Mostly we'd go on outings within the county.

Since I am an extraordinary group facilitator (I say that modestly), kids were encouraged to set the group's norms. This rule nailed me. Whatever the group votes to do is binding. To say Michael and Alan were fired up for the Lord is like saying Carter has liver pills. Unremittingly, they expressed their ideas and feelings about God and Jesus. Wouldn't you know it- they convinced the group to attend Alan's church. I was not thrilled. I didn't do church stuff.

The only time I had attended church was as a kid. On Easter Sunday, when I was around twelve years old, I went to church to get some Easter eggs and leave.. After I had my stuff, I quickly left. That particular Easter was the last time I saw any church, except for a funeral or two.

In accordance with the group's vote, one Friday we board a van for Grace Cathedral. It is a special church. Strange events take place there. Their pastor conducts miracle services and, coincidentally, they are held on Friday nights.

As the church comes into view I see a jammed parking lot. I openly wonder why it's so crowded. Someone remarked that people come from all over the country to get healed.

The Litmus Test

I remember thinking that this will be great. I'll put all this Jesus stuff to rest tonight because if the people don't get healed then all of this stuff is jive and I'll be done with it, Michael and Alan.

As we approach the greeter, strange but warm feelings overshadowed me. His relaxed and welcoming demeanor set me at ease. We took seats near the back. I saw the large stage and the wheelchair section off to the left near the front. I mostly notice that everyone there was white.

After we were seated, the usher sent a lady and a young man down our aisle to take seats next to me. Due to the narrowness of the row, they were forced to turn, face me, and shuffle sideways to their seats. The young man appeared to be in his late teens or early twenties and was sporting an unbuttoned shirt. As he slid past, the opened shirt revealed a large lump on his chest. I am pumped. This will be proof positive. This kid gets healed or he doesn't.

The healing service started and this young man moved to the front of the very long line. He finally made his way to the preacher. Like the others, he was struck on the forehead similar to the motion used to high five someone. However, in this case the forehead is smacked rather than the hand. His body went limp and one of the people placed to his rear caught him. He lay on the floor for several minutes and then he got up on his feet. I became very excited as he made his way back. He slid towards me. I could barely contain myself. The lady who came with him appeared anxious as well. She must know something that I don't. She screamed and burst into tears. Sliding by me the same way he did the first time, his chest is revealed to me. The lump was gone! All I could say is "Oh, no, oh, no, this stuff is real." I began to cry and couldn't stop. I placed my face into my hands. The kids kept asking if I was all right. I realized that my world would soon change drastically.

"What can I say?
Every mountain makes for tall ground
Boulders make a crash
Little pebbles make a small sound
Rebels make you bow down
I'm just a radical
Meaning I don't merely cheer for the King
I get fanatical"
Diicypulz—Mission, Movement, Music

CHAPTER 8

God's Draw

Although the experience at the church was undeniable, it didn't immediately alter my lifestyle of drinking, playing the ponies at various racetracks and playing poker with the fellows most Friday nights.

One rainy Friday night I headed up Route 8 to Northfield Park Racetrack. I didn't know much about thoroughbreds, let alone trotters and pacers, but that didn't diminish my thirst for action. While driving in the left lane I went to pass the car in front of me and to my right. I noticed the light at the intersection had just turned yellow. The driver of the car in the right lane slammed on his brakes and fishtailed in front of me. Instinctively, I veered left into the median. To my horror there were huge sewer pipes in the median only a couple of feet in front of me. My car was instantly lifted up over the pipes and placed on the road directly in front of the light. There were two other cars there—one was at the crossroad and the one that fishtailed. Both drivers and I just sat there incredulous for some time and then we all drove away.

Perhaps one day one of those individuals will read this and come forward. If they are at all like me, they know that there is a God somewhere who intervenes in the lives of people who don't even accept Him.

Did I give my heart to the Lord after this experience? No. Did I pause for a moment to thank God for his grace? No. I went on to the racetrack, but shortly after that I began to read a Bible.

"I bet you thought you killed me
But I'm back and wearing a crown
What don't kill me made me stronger
Now I've added some pounds
Bet you thought you had me scared
Bet you thought you had me there
But I found my purpose, I ain't worthless
Let me make it clear"
Diicypulz 2009

CHAPTER 9

Scared to Get Saved

Reading the Bible produced some peculiar emotions. Along with feelings of tremendous warmth, the words jumped out at me. Scriptures became believable. Actually, I began to believe the day the young man was healed, but this was different. I started to believe what the entire Bible revealed God and Jesus.

Michael, the kid from my group, held regular Bible studies. I made it my business to be there. I was pumped! I was motivated! I was ready to hear what thus sayeth the Lord and I wasn't even saved. One night Michael taught a lesson on the Holy Spirit. He shared his story of how he was at church praying and the Holy Spirit jumped on him and began to wrestle him. His face contorted as he explained this phenomenon. He said the Holy Spirit was all over him and held him down for a long time. This story stuck with me through my faith journey and I became more than a little concerned. Going WWE with the Holy Spirit, as a requirement for salvation, is a solemn predicament. You must remember, I had only been to church once in my life, and on that occasion I was merely there to get an Easter egg and leave. Slobbering all over myself while the Holy Spirit jacked me up in a full nelson was where I drew the line.

After my lesson on the Holy Spirit, I continued to read daily and my lifestyle changed. Drinking, gambling, and messing around with my girlfriend became history. I don't know if she really appreciated these changes, but I was trying to get something done.

The Desire for Salvation Consumed Me

Salvation was what I deeply desired. I honestly believed that Jesus had died, was buried, and was resurrected for my sins, but I was terrified of salvation. I didn't want the wrestling match. The Bible talks about confessing with your mouth the Lord Jesus but I hadn't done that.

A grand idea came to me. The pastor of that church where the young man received the miracle had a television show that aired regularly. I decided to watch the show and at the end I would confess Jesus as my Lord and Savior with all of the folks who went up for the invitation. Guess what? The show ended without an invitation.

My parade was postponed. I was crushed, despondent, disheartened—woe am I. Desperately wanting salvation but afraid to wrestle. I recall saying aloud, "I'm never going to get saved."

An Unconventional Approach to Salvation

Sensing the end of my spiritual tether was imminent; desperation plan number two was concocted. The intersection of Brittain Road and Tallmadge Avenue in Akron is very busy, especially at rush hour. You see where I am going? Think. What action do you take at a busy intersection at the height of rush hour if you want to enhance your chances of getting saved without a fight? Yep, my thought exactly. I waited at the intersection. My car was positioned first at the light. I thought that if the Holy Spirit wanted to wrestle with me and block all of this traffic, fine but I'm getting saved right here and right now!

Before the light turned green, I quickly recited a sinner's prayer. I looked around. Nothing. I listened and there was nothing. I'm ecstatic! I start shouting, "Praise God!" I'm saved and nothing has happened. I can't believe it. To me this was one of God's miracles, saved at last without a fight. How good is God?

People often remark how they would love to have supernatural experiences. I can understand that, but almost all of mine have been fairly frightening. In fact, after one that I will share later, I asked God not to give me anymore. He did not honor that request. People want more of God and want to experience more of His love. Some people just want to see something miraculous. I never did. I never prayed for these manifestations. I pray now only for power to help others in special ways. I really didn't need for God or His messengers to appear to me anymore.

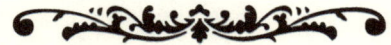

"If I could only get a glimpse of His face
Maybe a strand of hair
But I know the rules
I can't see Him until I land up there
Would I be clearing my throat to get my words straight?
Knowing just the feel of his cloak would set my nerves straight"
Diicypulz—Mission, Movement, Music

CHAPTER 10

I Learn My Mission

Now I'm saved. These supernatural manifestations should stop. There is no longer a need for a guy off the streets to be convinced that indeed there is a God. I could not have been more wrong. It happened one Saturday morning around10:00, as I recall. At that time, I lived in Barberton, Ohio with my Aunt Arcie. She was the proverbial gentle yet firm aunt that you seek out when a man born of a woman becomes full of trouble. I hated going to her when in desperate straits (broke). Her undivided attention never wavered. Invariably, she'd give me the money but not without the sermon. There would always be a sermon. The sermon highlights often did not include the Lord, just lessons about life and that awful word "responsibility".

After my Mom suffered a stroke, Aunt Arcie took Diane, Jerome, my Mom and myself into her home. Shortly thereafter my Mother succumbed to cancer.

Close Encounters of the God Kind

My aunt's barking dog interrupted my morning devotional. Morning meditations were not a habit. I just happened to be meditating over some Scriptures this particular morning. The sound of a barking dog echoed routinely, but this bark provoked a different feeling. It conveyed a warning. Had this occurred during the middle of the night I would have been more concerned; however, the daylight was reassuring.

As I lay on my right side the barking suddenly ceased. From my position I turned my head slightly to the left, looked up and saw this being. The manifestation revealed the form of a white outline of a man sketched into the bedroom door. There appeared an outline of something like hair on his head but I don't believe it was hair. I turned away not really grasping the magnitude of this vision. Then it hit me. There was something standing in the door. I don't mean in the doorway, I mean literally in the door!

I attempt. to look again but I am immediately paralyzed. I can only see a portion of the being, whatever you want to call him. Terrified does not even come close to conveying my fear. I could literally feel my skin crawl. Even though I knew I was in the presence of someone exceedingly powerful, I was determined to look fully at him. I said to myself, "I've got to see all of you." I try to turn with all of my might. Just then I heard the thundering voice that booms and echoes…No, Oh, Oh, Oh, Oh, Oh. It was like a thunderous wave…No, Oh, Oh, Oh, Oh, Oh. The sound shakes everything. I lay trembling. Every molecule in my body vibrated an uncontrollable frenzy.

What took place next defies logic. This coward of a person, me, stubbornly resolved to see him no matter what the cost. I say to myself again, "I have to see all of you." I try with all of my strength to turn to the left in order to see all of him. I'm released. The sheer force of my attempt rolls me completely out of the bed and onto the floor. Trembling, I look up and he's gone. I weep. I get on my knees and pray. Lord, I already believe. Please don't do this anymore. That very same voice answers, "Turn on the television." I said audibly, "Turn on the television?" I got up and turned it on. It was then that I noticed the time was 10:00. There is a show on at that time that features a young boy and an older gentleman with some sort of recreational vehicle. In any event, this kid is summoned to meet with a man in the clouds. This man gave him orders to assist someone on earth who is in dire need of help. The older guy takes the kid wherever he has been instructed to go. I watch two 15-minute episodes of this program. When it ends I turn off the television and return to my knees. The same voice (although now not audible, just in my mind) says, "Did you see how that young boy was sent to help people when they were in real need of help?" I say nothing. The voice goes on, "I'm going to use you in the same way. I am going to send you to people or people to you when they really need help."

I remained on my knees for quite awhile after that. Finally, I went into the living room. My aunt was there. I asked her if she had heard anything. She answered no. She heard only the bark of the dog.

Please know that the events that I share in this book are known only to a handful of people. These are individuals I have chosen to share them with or people who have witnessed them with me. This probably totals no more than twenty individuals.

You can't go around telling people you have seen angels or that God talks to you audibly. What will people think? I would not be writing this book now if God had not directed me to write it.

I will only share some of these events. I have decided to not include the evil forces that tried to stop me. I don't want to frighten readers nor do I feel led by God to do so.

I can hear you thinking, "Wow, this guy must be some kind of a super Christian. He must be really special". Honestly, I am not. I am just an ordinary believer.

Believe me- I have often wondered why God Almighty, the Great I AM, Creator of the universe, would bother with a person such as me.

Romans: 9 contained my answer. Paul's heart is filled with bitter sorrow and enduring grief for his fellow Jewish brothers and sisters. He was willing to be forever cursed—cut off from Christ—if that would save them.

Despite God revealing His glory to them, despite the covenants and special privileges of worship and receiving the promises reserved for them, despite their being chosen to be God's special children, they were not saved.

Paul writes, verses 6-13: Well then, has God failed to fulfill his promise to the Jews? No, for not everyone born into a Jewish family is truly a Jew! Just the fact that they are descendants of Abraham doesn't make them truly Abraham's children. For the Scriptures say, "Isaac is the son through whom your descendents will be counted," though Abraham had other children, too. This means Abraham's physical descendants are not necessarily children of God. It is the children of the promise who are considered to be Abraham's children. God had promised, "Next year I will return and Sarah will have a son."

This son was our ancestor Isaac. When he grew up, he married Rebecca, who gave birth to twins. But before they were born, before they had done anything good or bad, she received a message from God.

(This message proves that God chooses according to His own plan, not according to our good or bad works.) She was told, "The descendants of your older son will serve the descendents of your younger son." In the words of the Scriptures, "I loved Jacob, but I rejected Esau."

We are like Paul, wondering about God's fairness right here. God ends the speculation, "I will show mercy to anyone I choose, and I will show compassion to anyone I choose."

When God wants to conduct Kingdom business, He often uses the wind, rain, famine, angels, His word, animals, (particularly donkeys) and yes, you and me.

You would think that after all of these years, I would be some kind of preacher, pastor, bishop, anything but who I am. Like I said, I am nothing but a regular, ordinary guy that God Almighty chose to show things to and send on errands every now and again, those errands began right away.

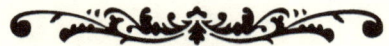

"You can tell by the smile that you see on me
That if you ever need a friend
You can lean on me
Hit the mall, hit the movie
Hit the scene on me
And we can both be who we gonna be"
Diicypulz—Mission, Movement, Music

CHAPTER 11

My Sister Diane

Growing up in a housing development (projects) with a mom who was often gone meant that Diane really raised my brothers and me. She did not care for this awesome responsibility. She and Mom argued often- and I mean they had some verbal slugfests. My delicate ears could hardly stand it. I was very nearly a model kid. I can't wait until Diane reads this. Diane was miffed...she could not understand why she had to baby-sit us so much. As a young teen she was responsible for three boys and herself on many occasions. Her activities were curtailed due to her position as reluctant mom.

I Harbor Deep Longings Regarding Her Mistreatments

For most of my adult life I have felt very sorry for my sister. She was never able to be a kid. Don't misunderstand me, she and I fought like most siblings. For her, abiding by the Geneva Convention was out of the question. Shoes, irons, and especially coke bottles were some of her favorite projectiles; The Cleveland Indians didn't possess an arm like hers. But still, I wished Mom had let her go hang out more.

As an adult I have tried to convey my love to her. I rarely tell her. I buy stuff for her. Hats delight her, especially those from Saks. How a poor girl developed such expensive taste is beyond me. She enjoys the compliments she gets while sporting them at church. I love seeing her face light up when she dons a new hat that I purchased. She used to keep the boxes.

Diane rebelled. At around age fourteen she could no longer take the restrictions so she up and left. I was devastated. She wasn't gone for very long, but it scared me to death. The etiology of my abandonment issues can be traced to her and that incident (I think).

Diane accepted the Lord shortly after I did. She mentioned that this intense light came into her room and did something to her. You'll have to ask her, but all I know is that she said she was saved. I witnessed her life begin to change. We started witnessing to people right there in the projects. We were on fire.

The same night of my morning visitation, Diane called me on the phone. It was late, after midnight. She said, "You need to come over here." I asked, "Why?" She said, "It's Marlene (fake name). I told her I would be right over. Barberton is about a 15 to 20 minute drive from North Akron. It seemed as if I made it in about three minutes.

Marlene always gave me the creeps. Even though we witnessed to her and she went to church with us, there was something sinister about her. I couldn't escape the feeling that she was the enemy. I'm not saying that she was.

The Holy Spirit

When I arrived at my sister's home, I walked right in. It was a warm summer night so Diane had the door open to allow the air to come through the screen door.

Upon entering, I saw Diane sprawled on the floor and looking terrified. Marlene was standing over her. When Marlene turned to look at me, my physical body sat down on the chair but I could see me standing up and shouting at her and praising God. Marlene ran out of the apartment.

Then my other body, being or whatever came back into me.

I stared off into space and my eyes welled up with tears as I revisited these events. I'm not sure what that was all about. Diane never could articulate what Marlene did to her. I just remember the voice. You know- the one that said he would send me to people or people to me when they really needed help,

These manifestations of our Lord are very hard to believe. I have often struggled wondering what people will think of me after reading these accounts. Lately my Bible opens to Psalm 73 almost every time I open it.

Being obedient I've read it in its entirety several times. The last time I read it the last verse jumped out at me.

Verse 28: But as for me, how good it is to be near God!
      I have made the Sovereign Lord my shelter,
      And I will tell everyone about the wonderful things you do.

"I tell em' that my life is the template
Set the pen, cutting through the madness like a tin blade
Shining like Edison, just to make it evident
Grateful, so at times I wanna' tithe about 7/10ths"
Diicypulz—Mission, Movement, Music

CHAPTER 12

Ahead

Would you believe there was a place drug users could go and learn all about the drugs they were about to ingest? They could learn of their overdose potential, classification, relative street value, and most importantly, what it could do for their head.

AHEAD also offered counseling services for individuals and families with alcohol and other drug problems. Its most used (abused) service was pill identification.

AHEAD is the acronym for Akron's House Extending Aid on Drugs. The house was purple. The idea being when a "head" (doper) was in trouble and needed to talk to another "head (lucent), they could call or walk into our very visible house; thus the name and the color.

Actually the term "head" took on a whole new significance. Many of the hired crisis intervention staff used drugs or alcohol or were "heads" themselves. Some even used drugs or alcohol while on the job or were high when arriving for work.

I Didn't Fit The Blueprint

Don't even ask me how I got hired. I applied for the job and they hired me. Was I a popular hire? Hardly. A non-using Christian in that environment was not realistic. The events that happened later proved that again it was God's will that I work there.

We provided services twenty-four/seven. Shift selection was simply genius. The supervisor would draw twenty-one rectangles on the board, each representing an eight-hour shift. By seniority, we'd pick rectangles, which contained a shift: midnight to 8, eight to four, or four to midnight. Somehow the five of us managed to cover the week.

In as much as I was the only Christian- oops- I mean, since I had the least amount of time in grade, I historically drew the worst shifts. I am talking about midnights and weekends. Working midnights presented some daunting challenges. You never knew who might walk through that door. A Dutch door separated us from whoever decided to walk in. The most challenging of all events was the chronic or constant caller.

Constant callers were people who were lonely. They called nearly every shift. We kept something called a constant callers log. The usual details were contained in the log and included the name of the caller, time, and general discussion. These callers mostly wanted company. One caller, a little lady with a raspy voice and a penchant for chain-smoking, whom I will call Ruby, called every shift. The midnight shift became her favorite. We talked a lot about music. Ruby played the guitar but she was musically challenged. That minor detail, however, never dissuaded her from asking me to listen.

One night I had Ruby and another constant caller on two lines. At those times I entertained thoughts of putting them both on hold, turning the phones upside down and letting them talk to each other. I never had the guts to do that but I heard of others doing it.

A Little Trickeration

Sometimes callers entertained suicidal ideation. With some of them I talked about the Lord. This did not go over very well with the dopers or the administration. A strong warning came my way to not speak about Jesus again.

This increased the number of callers who presented problems that were a lot more severe than normal. Some initiated discussions about Jesus. How subtle was that? Prior to the warning, not a single person had called to ask questions about Jesus. I had always broached the subject. Now folks were calling and wanting to know about Jesus. Coincidentally, it was only happening on my shift. I later learned that these callers were friends and acquaintances of the staff.

I didn't take the bait initially, but later on God began to let me know when I could share His love. He let me know when calls were authentic. I'd share his love and people would respond. Some would go back to their churches; some would accept Jesus as their Lord and Savior. Some attend my church to this day.

One night around 2 a.m. it was slow so I went into the living room and began to read my Bible. I heard someone out front so I slid my Bible under the chair. A white young man who appeared to be about twenty years of age walked into the foyer. I met him at the Dutch door and invited him in. He was slightly built and appeared distraught; I motioned for him to have a seat.

He accepted the invitation and uttered the only words he would for the entire visit: "Read to me from the Bible that you have under that chair." Sensing something special about him, I obeyed. The exact passages that I read escape me; however, the reading lasted a long time. After what seemed to be about an hour I asked if he wanted me to continue. He nodded. Tears streamed down his cheeks. He didn't bother to wipe them. I didn't bother to offer tissues. He never said a word. After reading for another half hour or so I stopped. He stood up, nodded his appreciation, and left.

God was sending people to me, or me to people when they really needed help. Although others came in late at night or early in the morning to talk, no other person ever identified the location of my Bible and directed me to read from it.

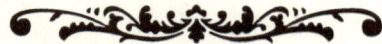

"They say the wise shall lead, but we need the young
And we can try all things underneath the sun
And never mind all things that we needed done
Being blind it just seems is the key to fun.
But somewhere along the line we depleted funds
And somewhere along with dying, old exceeded young
There's no sense in even trying if we see they won
There's no sense in even buying rather keep my one's"
Diicypulz-Mission, Movement, Music

Chapter 13

God Protects His Fools

In Ohio we like to say, "If you don't like the weather, give it twenty-four hours." The night was unusually warm for November. I wore only a fishnet shirt and slacks as I entered AHEAD for my midnight shift. At this time of year a sweater or coat would normally be worn.

My shift was uneventful, just the usual constant callers and pill identification. What became eventful was the dramatic change in weather. Overnight, wintry blizzard-like conditions set in. Cold, wind, and snow saluted me as I opened the door in preparation to leave.

I walked to work in those days. If I took the short cuts through the woods I could be home (my sister's apartment) in twenty minutes. Calling a cab was out of the question so I stuck it out. The wind chill was bone chilling. My breathing was labored and I was freezing. After just a couple of minutes I was forced to seek shelter. My fishnet shirt just wasn't cutting it.

The Mysterious Adventure Home

McDonald's was nearby so I ducked in there. The closest unoccupied table was all the way in the back of the restaurant. I was so cold that I went there and sat down. I didn't bother to go to the counter to order coffee. My fingers and toes were too numb to stand in line. I planned to order something to warm me up, but not just yet.

After a couple of minutes I noticed a tall white male standing at the counter. There was something awfully strange about this man. He was not dressed for winter—no hat, no coat, and no sweater. But even more noticeable was that his back was to the counter. He stood facing me and staring at me. He never turned around to order anything. Even more startling was that no one ever asked him if he wanted to order something. He stood gazing at me for the entire time I was there, which was probably eight to ten minutes.

I was not sitting particularly close to this man; I was near the back right side of the restaurant. The he spoke, "It's cold out there." His voice was in a normal tone but loud enough for me to hear. As he looked at me I nodded. He spoke again, "It's really cold out there." I said, "Yes, I know."

I kept wondering why none of the servers were asking him to order. He was taking up a lot of space at the counter but no one seemed to care or notice. No one even responded to his weather warnings except for me. He gave me one last warning, "It's cold out there." I nodded again.

A few minutes later I walked out of McDonald's to continue the journey home. I passed by him on my way out the door. He just looked at me. Outside it felt much colder. My bones were cold. Just a couple of minutes beyond McDonald's was a bowling alley. The sharp, cold wind forced me to seek shelter there. No one was there but a short, portly, white lady at the counter. By now it was about 8:30 in the morning. I got some coffee and took a table. I was there about twenty minutes and went out again. This time I was determined to make it all the way to my sister's home.

Running across Market Street, I decided to take a short cut through Grace Park. It's a small park nestled between Market and Perkins Streets. I took the shortcut down Summit Street, which is a fairly steep hill that intersects Furnace Street at the bottom. I ran over the railroad tracks, through the woods, and down to Spring Street. Spring Street was a narrow street that ran under the old viaduct (bridge). It was notorious for catching jumpers who saw fit to end their life. As kids, whenever word spread that someone had jumped off the bridge we'd all go running up Spring Street to see the body. I never saw a body. The police had always scooped them up before I could get there. I honestly didn't want to see the mangled bodies. Peer pressure beat me to death so I wimped out probably like many of the other kids.

My strength was holding up as I left the park and reached Furnace Street. Running down the street kept me warm. At the bottom of the street were railroad tracks that ran parallel to Furnace Street. It was at this location that I heard the voice. The voice was very loud and very clear. It roared, "What are you running for?" Stopping dead in my tracks, I turned, looked up at the top of Furnace Street and saw the same guy who was at the counter in McDonald's. I'm incredulous…I think, *"What is wrong with this guy?"* He again just stood there. I was so cold, trembling now. I took off across the tracks and down a trail through the woods and onto Spring Street.

Now I was in huge trouble. My pace slowed to a point that I could barely move. I had no feeling in my leg, or hands…I thought I was going to die right there where those jumpers entered eternity. Then, miraculously, a stream of warm air engulfed me. I was warm all over. I started to run again. I ran the remainder of the way to my sister's apartment assisted by this gentle stream of warm air. I knocked on the door. My sister opened and looked at me in total astonishment. She had a few choice words for me for being so stupid to come that far in weather not fit for man or beast. She could not believe that all I had on was a fishnet shirt.

She directed my attention to the television. The news anchor was reporting on the number of people who were being seen at emergency rooms for frostbite. I suffered neither frostbite nor any other complication from my ordeal. I knew why I was okay. I kept thinking about that man in McDonald's. He was the same guy who yelled at me from the top of Furnace Street. A man who was dressed with not much more clothing than me. A man who stood with his back to the counter yet never ordered and was never asked to order. A man sent by God to protect a fool. Praise God.

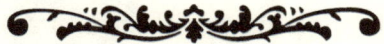

"Sometimes, just to give them all that they need makes it a long night.
Praying that we don't have to bleed within the long fight.
Gave em' just the person they've seen within their own eyes.
Maybe if we gave em' the seams, they'd put us on tight.
It doesn't really matter; we're only here for the King's praise.
Real enough to finally make it beyond your ten plays?"
Diicypulz-Sophomore Project

CHAPTER 14

Who's That Lady?

One evening I lay in bed relaxing to the rhythmic taps of rain pounding on my roof and awning. I gaze at the clock noting the time, 8:45 p.m. Turning in early is unusual for me but this particular evening I felt like resting.

For reasons unbeknownst to me and even though it was getting late, I had an intense desire to go to Kaufmann's Department Store. As bizarre as this seems, I rationalized that I did not have a dress belt and now would be a good time to go and get it. The store closed at 10:00 p.m. thus providing ample time to accomplish this mission.

An Offer I Could Have Refused

I got myself out and headed for the door. Wow, what a deluge outside, but out I went. Backing out of the drive and heading up the street, I only went about ten yards. I noticed a white woman was walking towards me. I was amazed anyone would be out walking in this weather. She approached my car and motioned for me to the lower the window. She asked if I was going to the southeast side of town. I told her, "No, I'm heading north towards Montrose." It is obviously almost the direct opposite of her destination.

I raised the passenger side window and pulled away. I watched her in my rearview mirror. Only a flimsy hand held piece of plastic held over her head protected her from the downpour. Feeling compassion for her, I stopped my car. In an instant she was at my door and let herself in. We discussed her intentions very specifically with regard to where she was headed.

During the trip I learned that she provided care for an elderly man. We were headed to his home. She said he was there alone and needed her assistance. When I asked her about her car, she said it broke down near my house and the tow truck driver wanted twenty-five dollars to tow it. She didn't have the money so he refused to tow it. That's when she started walking. I asked her if she wanted me to give her the money and she didn't respond. I gave it to her anyway.

Driving Miss Lady

While driving on the freeway I couldn't help but notice all of the standing water. I drove exceedingly slow due to the conditions. She directed me to a side street that was off of Arlington Street. She pointed to a house and said that was where she was going. I pulled up and stopped in front of the house on the far side of the street, which required her to walk around my car and cross the street to get to the house.

The street was not at all lit. The house was totally dark. I asked if the guy was in the house. She assured me he was. After thanking me profusely she opened the door and walked to the back of the car. I turned my head to the left to watch her walk across the street. Guess what? She was not there. She had vanished into thin air; there was no sign of her. In an instant she was gone. In the time it took me to turn my head she was nowhere to be seen. I got out of my car and looked for her but it was to no avail. I gazed intently at the house. The lights never came on.

I have no idea what this encounter was all about. All I know is that the angel told me that I would be sent to people or people to me when they really needed help.

Needless to say I never made it to the store to get that belt. This encounter produced nothing but questions:

- Who was that lady?
- Why did God send me out in a downpour for a chance encounter for no apparent reason?
- If this lady was an angel, do the same laws in the flesh bind them as they are in heaven and the spirit world? Can angels lie to get you to accomplish something?

- Was God trying to show me how easily He can change the direction of our lives?

- Remember…I was going to purchase a belt.

My question for you is, "What do you do with unexplained spiritual phenomena?"

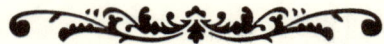

"I can't wait just to hear the applause, while walking through the gates.
Take a little bow and pause, to look at all the greats.
And finally see the Man, I wrapped my whole life around.
I'll probably ask my Savior for some paper, just to write it down."
Diicypulz—The Sophomore Project

CHAPTER 15

The Triple Digits

A radio with a digital clock rests on a table beside my bed. The numbers on the clock are red. For whatever reason(s) I rarely sleep through the night. Getting eight hours of sleep has escaped me for as long as I can remember. I have acculturated to tossing and turning and getting up to relieve myself while most folks are snoring or making other benign noises.

Encounters of the Numerical Kind

Slowly it begins to happen. I'd awaken to make my nightly traipse to the bathroom but I'd notice these red numbers on the clock in triple digits. The clock would read 333, 444, or 555, whenever I would wake up and look at the radio. Because I sleep on my right side, I would awaken and turn left and observe the numbers. At first I didn't pay much attention. Then it became more and more noticeable. For weeks I'd awaken at exactly one of the triple digits, usually 555. Every night for weeks I'd awaken, roll over, look at the radio and see triple red digits.

During one of these episodes, I got on my computer and emailed my Bishop, Joey Johnson. To my surprise a response came that very morning from him while I was still up surfing the net. He mentioned he thought God was trying to get my attention. In response, every time I awakened to triple digits I went into my prayer closet (living room in front of my couch) and prayed. Often during those times of prayer I would be frightened and feel as if God was protecting me from something or someone. At other times I engaged in a worship experience that lifted my soul nearly out of my house. The power of God would sometimes rest upon me.

Often I'd experience a peace that went beyond description. I can only describe it as overwhelming warmth that gently bends you into a fetal position and rocks you with undulating waves of warmth.

Because of these encounters I started a devotional hour at 10:00 p.m. nightly. It was during one such devotional that Jesus gave me this message of hope.

"We'd rather focus on who's making money and who isn't
But the one's making something still are lacking vision.
Maybe that shows money ain't the only answer
Cause money can't give life when you're given cancer.
In the grand scheme- you don't have a friend then you can't lean
Life without love's like a bad dream
Or the naked one
In school where you're naked running down the hallway while they're
making fun."
Diicypulz 2009

CHAPTER 16

Let It Rage!

Why do the heathen rage and the people imagine a vain thing?

Sometimes God asks us questions. These are special times. On these occasions he lends his undivided attention.

Why does an omniscient God question mere mortals? Let's just say he is the ultimate therapist. As any ultimate therapist would do, he leads the session with a question. He grants an opportunity to unload, to pour out, and to vent our troubles.

Indulge me for a minute.

Intermittent Explosive Disorder

Were you aware that there is a seldom-studied mental illness that deals with rage? Meet Intermittent Explosive Disorder, an illness characterized by recurrent episodes of angry and potentially violent outbursts. It's seen mainly in cases of road rage or spousal abuse and has been found to be much more common than previously thought.

How about that? Intermittent Explosive Disorder. In any event, it affects 16 million Americans in their lifetime, reports Ronald Kessler, Ph.D., a professor of health care policy at Harvard Medical School (HMS) and his colleagues.

Intermittent Explosive Disorder attacks are out of proportion to the social stressors triggering them and are not due to another mental disorder or the effects of drugs or alcohol, according to the Diagnostic and Statistical Manual of Mental Disorders, Fourth Edition (DSM-IV). People with this disorder overreact to situations with uncontrollable rage, feel a sense of relief during the angry outburst, and then feel remorseful about their actions.

See, that's why as much as possible with my fleshy self, I try to get along with folks. You never know what kind of day a person is encountering. Since Intermittent Explosive Disorder attacks are out of proportion to the stressors causing them, people are subject to show you their middle finger—or worse—with little provocation.

William J. Cromie of the Harvard News Office, in an article entitled, Anger Can Break Your Heart, writes, "Think about this the next time someone cuts you off in traffic or in a grocery store line: anger can bring on a heart attack or stroke."

Men Had Better Watch Out

That's the conclusion of several studies at Harvard Medical School and elsewhere. One study of 1,305 men with an average age of 62, revealed that the angriest men were three times more likely to develop heart disease than the most placid ones.

Angry older men, as stereotypes go, are most vulnerable. But excessive ire can take a toll at any age.

"Almost all the anger research I'm familiar with has focused on men," notes Simon. "However, based on a 2006 study of road rage, I would guess that women are less prone to severe anger and thus to its deleterious effects, which include heart attack, stroke, and even impaired lung function."

Wait a minute. So far all of these findings seem right on. But it's obvious these guys don't get out much. I know some women who, when angry, will tear a man or beast a new hide. Once I knew a woman who was reputed to be the most vicious person in our housing development (project). During one altercation she lifted a man in the air and launched him over a three-foot bridge and into the canal that ran under it. The poor man fell about ten feet. She was never arrested. I think the police were afraid to come get her.

And what of the volumes written about hell and fury and women scorned?

My unofficial research (life experience) suggests both women and men suffer from Intermittent Explosive Disorder. They just manifest it differently. Women seem to internalize it and wait for the right moment to strike back, while men just let it rip and vomit their rage all over everyone.

Simon suggests learning to meditate, or experimenting with deep breathing exercises to stay cool. He goes on to say, "Don't boil in silence. Talk out your feelings with your spouse, partner, or a good friend. If that doesn't work, write down your feelings, and try to explain to yourself why you are so irritated or vexed."

God's Remedy For Rage Is Contained In The Psalms

In The Bible, the book of Psalms contains many different types of psalms. Some are referred to as psalms of Thanksgiving; others are about kings or enthronement psalms. Still others are about wisdom. There are many more but the most popular type of psalm is one of lament. Folks cry and complain about God's lack of attention to a pressing need. Needs like food, shelter, and oh, by the way, we are about to die if you don't hurry up and do something about these approaching heathens.

God's timing is amazing. Often he inquires of us when our lives are up for grabs. I call it spiritual despondency. I know that feeling more intimately than I should. You might know it also. It's when life isn't turning out the way you planned. Your gut has turned jelly-like from all of life's poundings. You feel trapped by nightmarish thoughts. Spiritual goals have vanished. What was once a raging river of enthusiasm for God's Word has become an annoying drip of despair.

In my case my financial empire crumbled like the walls of Jericho. Hope was shattered. In the past, fervent study of God's Word yielded wonderful messages. I'd see myself preaching. My messages would inspire, encourage, and stimulate. Now, messages seemed empty, encouraging thoughts went AWOL and my evil twin stimulated no one.

Before spiritual despondency, I looked forward to meeting new people and developing new friendships, but while in its grip I only hung with people I liked and who liked me, too.

I was stuck. My decisions sucked. I was miserable, though I didn't approach the depths of Job's misery by a long shot.

God impressed a question upon me. Maybe He was granting me an audience, much like he did for Job. Let's take a look at Job.

Job had a mountain of problems. He was a mountain of a man who lived in the land of Uz. He was blameless and a man of honor. He feared God and steered clear of evil. He had a nice family consisting of seven sons and three daughters. He owned hundreds of animals and employed many servants. He was, in fact, the richest person in the entire area.

Notice the integrity of Job. Every year when Job's sons had birthdays, they invited their brothers and sisters to join them for a celebration. On these occasions they would get together to eat and drink. When these celebrations ended—and sometimes they lasted for several days—Job would purify his children by getting up early in the morning and presenting a burnt offering for each of them. This was just in case they had sinned overtly or even considered the thought. Job said to himself, "Perhaps my children have sinned and have cursed God in their hearts." I don't know about you but my experience with drinking, eating, and partying is that somebody almost always partakes of a little sin. In any case, *preparing "just in case" burnt offerings* was Job's regular practice.

Things were going well for Job. God was even bragging on him. He asked Satan, "Have you noticed my servant Job? He is the finest man in all of the earth—a man of complete integrity. He fears God and will have nothing to do with evil."

A Supernatural Test

Satan replied to the Lord, "Yes, Job fears God, but not without good reason! You have always protected him, and his home, and his property from harm. You have made him prosperous in everything he does. Look how rich he is! But take away everything he has, and he will surely curse you to your face!"

The test was on. God granted Satan permission to test Job but with one condition. "Do whatever you want with everything he possesses, but don't harm him physically." Job's first test started ominously. A messenger arrived at Job's home with this news: "Your oxen were plowing, with the donkeys feeding beside them, when the Sabeans raided us. They stole all of the animals and killed all the farmhands. I am the only one who escaped to tell you."

While this guy was still speaking another guy arrived with the news that the fire of God had fallen down from heaven and burned up Job's sheep and all the shepherds. Just like the first messenger, he was the only one who escaped to tell Job.

Would you believe that another messenger arrived? He said, "Three bands of Chaldean raiders have stolen your camels and killed your servants. I am the only one who escaped to tell you."

You Won't Believe This But...

Yet while he was speaking, another messenger arrived with the news: "Your sons and daughters were feasting in their older brother's home. Suddenly a powerful wind swept in from the desert and hit the house on all sides. The house collapsed and all of your children are dead. I am the only one who escaped to tell you."

Job stood up, tore up his robe in grief. He shaved his head and fell to the ground before God. He said, "I came into this world naked and I'll be naked when I die. The Lord gave me everything I had, and the Lord has taken it away. Praise the name of the Lord! In all this Job did not blame God.

That Was Only The First Test

For his second test Satan received permission from God to take away Job's health. He struck Job with a terrible case of boils that completely obscured his body. Job scraped his skin with a piece of broken pottery as he sat among the ashes. It got so bad that his wife said to him, "Are you still trying to maintain your integrity? Curse God and die."

But he wouldn't. He said, "Should we accept only the good things from God and never anything bad?" So still, Job did nothing wrong.

If Job had stopped right there he would have been fine. But he didn't. He had a few things on his mind and body. There was much he wanted to get off his chest. Indeed he did. He cursed the day of his birth.

Again, my distressing situation was not on par with Job's, but just as puppy love is love to puppies, my spiritual dispossession was agonizing to me. I had some thoughts to get off my chest as well.

It was at this time during one of my devotionals that I felt the Lord asking me, "Why do the heathens rage and the people imagine a vain thing?

I unloaded. Maybe it's because the very first person you died for was a blood thirsty, sadistic murderer named Barrabas. What kind of a message is that? What are people supposed to think? Why should they bother getting saved? They can do their dirt. They can savage one another sexually. They can exploit systems and people for material gain. They can go on boasting about the superiority of their race, family, education, kids, their economic status and so forth and so on. Then when finally satisfied they can sheepishly come to you, ask forgiveness and be saved. And you are going to save them.

Lord even when people were deriding you on the cross you said, "Father, forgive them for they know not what they do."

So they continued to rage and imagine vain things.

They Rage Due To Injustices

Maybe it's because they lost both parents before age twenty. Their mom probably died a slow, painful death due to complications from a stroke and cancer. Their father more than likely checked into a hospital with a minor problem. He ended up dying of gangrene and other medical problems that one could never understand. And everywhere they looked, they saw injustices. They see pimps, prostitutes, street hustlers, corporate hustlers, child molesters and more. People who represent the worst of society are alive and well. Some are even thriving, yet their parents who were decent people are dead. How is that fair?

And so they rage.

Heathens are probably upset over college girls. I am talking about those lying college girls who profess Christianity. I've spotted them strutting around campus expressing how they love the Lord. Yet they sleep around. They are rather sleazy, rather regularly. They're nothing but easy prey, easily trading their values like a commodities broker.

How about this? These heathens hated Christians. As far as they were concerned Christians were a bunch of excessively servile and obedient fools who believe in a white man's God. But through the work of others and the Holy Spirit, you drew them to you with supernatural love. For the first time in a long time they were hopeful that there is a God who loved them and had a plan for their life. Supplied with that expectation they walked right off the street and into a church. They were filled with a desire to learn more of your love and embrace those who love you.

But because they were wearing jeans and a fishnet shirt and a little sweat, no such love was found- only unwelcome glances and stares. They turned their back on that church and left. They kept on raging.

They also see divorced Christians struggling with skin hunger while not being able to marry again unless they get reconciled to their ex. That ex who just happens to be remarried. Who wants a life like that? Even heathens know that a man can't go the rest of his life without sex. I'll bet you that is why they are raging. Maybe they are nice people who grew weary giving their lives for others. Do you know what happened in Mark, Chapter 6? The disciples had just completed a long missionary journey and they were going on about all that happened when you mentioned everyone should find some rest. You went somewhere and still were confronted with vast crowds. Even the disciples were weary and needed rest and wanted you to send the people away. So how do you think these heathens feel when they become tired and exasperated? They want to quit.

Church Service And Brother Harris

I remember a church service to commemorate our new sanctuary. I was feeling just like these heathens…tired of people. I was tired of listening to their problems, tired of giving them money, tired of giving them food, and just plain tired of just being there for them. At the beginning of the service Bishop Johnson asked everyone to form prayer groups. During our group prayer I expressed my annoyance with people. I was tired and wasn't going to help anyone else…ever! I had never offered a prayer like that before but I did then. The others prayed and we broke for a service of celebration. The celebration did not mitigate my misery. After service I ran into Brother Harris. He is a big man who usually offers a very warm greeting. Tonight was no exception. "Hey, *Dan the Man*, how are you?" Before I could reply he went on, "I had this dream about you." I thought, "Oh no." With the way I had been feeling, I braced for the worst. He said, "Man it was a great dream. You were helping all these people." He gave me one of those big bear hugs and an understanding smile. I made an excuse to leave and walked away. After a few paces I could not stop the tears.

See Lord, you are going to keep sending people to me for help and you are going to make me keep helping them. It doesn't matter how much they take advantage of me or abuse my acts of kindness. I'm going to have to just keep on helping them. Heathens know of this and wonder why you do that.

That's why they're raging and that's why they imagine a vain thing.

God's Response

I got that off my chest and I felt better. What did God do? He listened to my complaint and sent me on a mission to help someone else.

Does God accept this whining and complaining? Yes, He even seems to encourage it. After all, counselors know that crying and complaining is a cathartic release.

According to a Harvard business study, rage affects one out of ten men and one out of twenty women. The study doesn't tell you what to do about it.

When I was counseling and a new client came through the door, I could start a new session without reading the client's intake form. I would start my session with a question and 90% of the time I would be right on target. The question was, "Who are you angry with?" I used that tactic twenty years ago.

What does this say to us? There are way too many angry folks walking around.

Let me share something. Hold on to your breastplate because you are going to be pleasantly surprised. You might have a spiritual gift that you knew nothing about.

First, take a look at this Psalm and see if you can see the gift I'm referring to.

Psalm 142:
With my voice I cry to the Lord;
With my voice I make my supplication to the Lord.
I pour out my complaint before Him;
I tell my trouble before Him.

Of course you see it. It's the gift of complaining. Okay, maybe it's not one of the spiritual gifts. However, if you can complain with the best of them, you might be closer to God than you think. Now I would focus on complaining to God and not to your friends and neighbors.

People become annoyed with moaning and groaning very quickly. They lack an appreciation for that sort of thing.

God Sends Kate

I have had the opportunity to share this message a couple of times. I would describe the first opportunity that arose as simply astounding. I was having a recurring dream. About once every three months it would visit. It was the most blissful dream ever. In this dream I am roller-skating. (I skate on quads. Blades are not for me.) I absolutely loved this dream. While skating, I perform an array of jaw dropping moves. You've seen commercials where skydivers perform spins, back flips, front flips and the like. Well, in my dreams I do the same things while weightless. I'm in a small gym. There are lots of other skaters, mainly kids. While floating up and down and spinning sideways, I come amazingly close to the floor, but then I accomplish an acrobatic move to gently lift me up again.

In any event, the evening following the last dream, I attended our Wednesday church service. After service, like many folks, I hung around hugging, greeting, and exchanging pleasantries. I looked up to see Kate Beggs approaching me. Her face beamed. Kate was one of my young tennis instructors. What came out of her mouth was truly astonishing. "Coach Dan, I would really love to go skating but I don't have anyone to go with." I didn't know what to say. I hadn't skated regularly in years, about forty to be exact.

Since thoughts of the dream warmed me, I agreed to meet her at the rink.

We met at the North Canton Skate Center to do our thing. Getting back into skating was daunting but I managed. I even enjoyed myself so I went a few more times.

God Sends Sister Mae

One night, as I skated slowly around the rink, a lady approached me. She said her name was Sister Mae. She went on to tell me that she was a pastor of a small church in Canton, Ohio. Then she said, "I would like for you to come and speak at my church." This woman did not know me. I declined. I told her I was not a preacher and besides, I had no message. She replied, "God will give you a message," and she skated away. I gave it some thought and decided God has given me a message. I cut across the rink and caught up to her. I told her God had in fact already given me a message. We made arrangements for me to speak at her church. I spoke there about a month later and shared the message Jesus gave me. It was glorious.

"Feel like I'm in a love affair with my king
And I can't help but share what I've seen
'Cause nothing can compare to this thing
It's so amazing, His love is so amazing.
Feel like I'm in a love affair with my king
And I can't help but stand up and sing
I need it like the air that I breathe
And so I'm taking, His love has got me takin'"
Diicypulz 2009

CHAPTER 18

When Life Has Your Number
(Or When Keeping the Faith Doesn't Work)

I'm standing three feet from her desk with my fists clenched, nostrils flared, and eyes piercing. All of the muscles in my body are poised to erupt. Whey wouldn't she just take the money? The sign on the wall behind and above her head read Chima Travel. She is professional and warm, the kind of assistant that every employer covets.

She was a woman exuding virtue, whose eyes convey understanding, acceptance, and empathy. I noticed her long, slender, white fingers with well-manicured nails coated in a clear polish. She was classy. She collected and stacked the money with the adroitness of a Las Vegas card dealer. Bills in small denominations are scattered all over her desk. I can't believe her calm demeanor. Why doesn't she call 911? Why doesn't she buzz her boss for assistance with this irate black man who (in a fit of rage) just threw a huge stack of money at her? Could she possibly know how much I hurt? Could she know that I had spent the last few nights lying prostrate on the floor weeping and convulsing in a pool of tears?

Could she know that I am the proverbial mental health professional whose life is a mess? Yet, I am obligated to reassure clients of the possibilities of each new day.

She couldn't know my shades at home stay pulled, curtains remain closed, and the phone remains off the hook.

Most important, she doesn't know I have had it with my lot in life. I was off to Las Vegas to launch my new career…that of a professional gambler. No more of this faith stuff for me. Like Peter going back to his fishing career after the crucifixion of Jesus, I was dumping this life and making a new start. That's why I am at Chima Travel, standing in front of this sales assistant.

The only thing between a new life and me was this woman. She booked my trip. I had the flight, the hotel, a rental car, and a new lease on life. I was all set until she asked for my credit card. I put my right hand in my back pocket...nothing. I placed both hands, palms down, on two front pockets. To my relief I found lots of cash. It was much more than I needed to pay for this trip. A couple of my tenants had paid their rent in cash. I offered to pay for the entire trip with cash. She declined and insisted that I pay with a credit card. She said they had to use my credit card to reserve the room and rental car. I paused, froze, and thought, "Where is my wallet?"

I searched my pockets again to no avail. I became incensed and flung all of my cash all over her desk and screamed, "Take it."

Silence ensued. Slowly and without a word she collected the money. She told me politely that she would gladly help me later today or tomorrow when I brought in my credit card.

Feeling Pretty Low

She handed me the bills. I accepted them with regret and headed for home. Once home, I conducted a frantic search for my wallet. I wanted to find it immediately and head back to Chima Travel. I ransacked my house, turning it inside out in search of that wallet. Yet it was not to be found.

The next morning like the prodigal son, I regained my senses. I got up early to prepare for the day. When I was walking towards the bathroom, I noticed an object on my dining room table. Lord have mercy, it's my wallet!

To this day I have no idea how that wallet got there. There is usually nothing on my table. I'll leave it up to you to draw your own conclusions.

Let me ask you a question. What is faith? The usual response is that faith is the substance of things hoped for and so on. Faith is active and what you do without clear proof. Those answers are good.

Consider what Paul said, "I have kept the faith." Consider what my dying friend said just a few days before he died...."tell them I have kept the faith." Do you see what faith is? Faith is something you keep. God is so good that sometimes he will help you keep it. He might even hide your wallet.